CONTENTS

Introduction 1

Chapter one 5

Chapter Two 8

Chapter Three 13

Chapter Four 21

Chapter Five 44

Chapter 6 50

Conclusion 54

INTRODUCTION

Exploring the Carnivore Diet

The Carnivore Diet has gained significant attention in recent years as a dietary approach that stands in stark contrast to conventional nutrition wisdom. In this exploration, we'll delve into the core principles of the Carnivore Diet, its potential benefits, and its controversies.

Understanding the Carnivore Diet

The Carnivore Diet is a highly restrictive dietary plan that revolves around one primary principle: the exclusive consumption of animal products. This includes meat, fish, and animal-derived products like eggs and dairy. The central idea is to eliminate all plant-based foods, such as fruits, vegetables, grains, and legumes. Advocates of this diet argue that humans evolved as carnivores and that by returning to this ancestral diet, one can achieve optimal health.

Key Principles

1. **Exclusivity**: The Carnivore Diet strictly prohibits the consumption of plant-based foods. Followers believe that this eliminates potential allergens and anti-nutrients found in plants, leading to improved health.

2. **Animal-Based Nutrition**: The diet relies on nutrient-dense animal foods, such as red meat and organ meats, to provide essential vitamins, minerals, and protein.

3. **Zero Carbohydrates**: Carbohydrates are almost entirely eliminated from the diet, with the exception of trace amounts found in animal products.

4. **Fat Emphasis**: Fat is a significant component of the Carnivore Diet, often comprising the majority of daily caloric intake. This includes both animal fat and saturated fats.

Why the Carnivore Diet is Effective for Weight Loss

The effectiveness of the Carnivore Diet for weight loss has been a topic of debate and fascination. Advocates claim that this diet can lead to rapid weight loss and improved body composition. Let's delve into the mechanisms behind these purported benefits.

Ketosis and Weight Loss

One of the primary reasons the Carnivore Diet is believed to promote weight loss is its induction of ketosis. Ketosis occurs when the body switches from using glucose as its primary energy source to burning fat for fuel. Since the diet is extremely low in carbohydrates, the body starts breaking down stored fat for energy, resulting in weight loss.

Reduced Appetite

The high-fat content of the Carnivore Diet can also contribute to reduced appetite. Fat is known for its satiating properties, which means that individuals on this diet may feel fuller for longer periods, reducing overall caloric intake.

Insulin Sensitivity

Another potential benefit is improved insulin sensitivity. By eliminating carbohydrates, the diet may help stabilize blood sugar levels and reduce insulin spikes. Improved insulin sensitivity can lead to better control over hunger and cravings, ultimately aiding in weight loss.

Elimination of Processed Foods

The Carnivore Diet's strict guidelines often lead to the elimination of processed and junk foods. This alone can result in weight loss as individuals are no longer consuming high-calorie, low-nutrient items that contribute to weight gain.

Controversies and Considerations

It's important to note that while some people may experience significant weight loss on the Carnivore Diet, it is not without controversies and potential drawbacks. The diet's long-term sustainability, nutrient deficiencies, and concerns about its impact on heart health have raised significant questions among healthcare professionals.

The Importance of a Well-Balanced Cookbook

In a world where countless diets and dietary preferences exist, the need for a well-balanced cookbook cannot be overstated. Such a cookbook serves as a valuable resource for individuals looking to maintain a balanced and nutritious diet while exploring different culinary traditions.

Variety and Nutrition

A well-balanced cookbook offers a diverse range of recipes that incorporate various food groups, including fruits, vegetables, lean proteins, and whole grains. This variety ensures that individuals receive a wide spectrum of nutrients necessary for overall health.

Cultural Exploration

Cookbooks that feature recipes from different cultures provide an opportunity for culinary exploration. This not only adds excitement to meal preparation but also exposes individuals to a world of flavors and cooking techniques that can be both enjoyable and nutritious.

Dietary Accommodations

A well-balanced cookbook should also cater to dietary restrictions and preferences. This includes recipes suitable for vegetarians, vegans, gluten-free diets, and more. Inclusivity in a cookbook ensures that everyone can find dishes that align with their unique dietary needs.

Meal Planning and Preparation

Cookbooks often include meal planning guides and tips for efficient meal preparation. These resources can be invaluable for busy individuals looking to maintain a balanced diet while managing a hectic schedule.

Encouraging Home Cooking

Perhaps one of the most significant advantages of a well-balanced cookbook is its potential to encourage home cooking. Preparing meals at home allows individuals to have greater control over ingredients, portion sizes, and cooking methods, ultimately contributing to better health outcomes.

CHAPTER ONE

Understanding the Carnivore Diet

The Carnivore Diet: A Deep Dive

The Carnivore Diet has garnered a significant amount of attention in recent years for its unconventional approach to nutrition. This diet, characterized by its extreme restriction of plant-based foods and exclusive focus on animal products, has generated both fascination and controversy. In this exploration, we will delve into the origins, key principles, misconceptions, and myths surrounding the Carnivore Diet.

What is the Carnivore Diet?

The Carnivore Diet, also known as the all-meat diet, is a dietary regimen that revolves around the consumption of animal-based foods exclusively. This means that individuals following this diet avoid all plant-based foods, including fruits, vegetables, grains, nuts, and seeds. The primary staples of the Carnivore Diet are typically beef, pork, poultry, fish, and other animal products like eggs and dairy.

Key Principles and Rules to Follow

1. Animal-Based Exclusivity: The most fundamental principle of the Carnivore Diet is to consume only animal-based foods. Followers of this diet argue that humans are biologically adapted to thrive on animal products and that plants should be entirely eliminated from the diet.

2. Zero Carbohydrate Intake: Another key rule is the elimination of carbohydrates. This includes avoiding not only refined sugars and grains but also healthy carb sources like fruits and vegetables. The idea is to keep carb intake as close to zero as possible.

3. Emphasis on Fatty Cuts: Advocates of the Carnivore Diet recommend focusing on fatty cuts of meat. This preference for fatty meats is driven by the belief that fat provides a more efficient source of energy than carbohydrates.

4. Minimal Seasoning: The Carnivore Diet promotes minimalism when it comes to seasoning. Salt is usually allowed, but spices, herbs, and other condiments are discouraged.

5. Water and Salt: Adequate hydration is essential, and followers are encouraged to drink water as needed. Additionally, salt intake is emphasized to prevent electrolyte imbalances.

The History and Origins of the Diet

The Carnivore Diet, though gaining recent popularity, is not a new concept. Its historical origins can be traced back to various indigenous populations and explorers who survived on animal-based diets out of necessity. One notable example is the Inuit people of the Arctic, who traditionally subsisted mainly on fish and marine mammals.

In contemporary times, the diet gained renewed attention through the work of individuals like Dr. Shawn Baker and Dr. Paul Saladino, both of whom advocate for the health benefits of an all-meat diet. The modern resurgence of the Carnivore Diet can be attributed to the growth of the low-carb and high-fat diet movements, which overlap with some aspects of this diet.

Common Misconceptions and Myths

As with any dietary approach, the Carnivore Diet has its fair share of misconceptions and myths. Let's address some of the most prevalent ones:

1. Lack of Nutrients: Critics often argue that the diet lacks essential nutrients found in plant-based foods, such as vitamins, fiber, and antioxidants. However, proponents of the Carnivore Diet contend that animal products provide all necessary nutrients in sufficient quantities.

2. Digestive Issues: Concerns about digestive problems due to the absence of fiber are common. While some individuals may experience an adjustment period, proponents argue that the digestive system adapts to an all-meat diet over time.

3. High Risk of Heart Disease: The high saturated fat content of many animal products has led to concerns about heart health. Supporters of the diet point to studies suggesting that saturated fat may not be as harmful as once thought and that the absence of carbohydrates can improve certain cardiovascular risk factors.

4. Long-Term Sustainability: Critics question the long-term sustainability of the Carnivore Diet. They argue that excluding a wide range of foods may lead to deficiencies and health issues over time. Proponents, however, often cite anecdotal evidence of improved health and well-being.

CHAPTER TWO

Benefits of the Carnivore Diet

Weight Loss and Fat Burning

Weight loss and fat burning are topics that have garnered significant attention in recent years due to the growing awareness of the importance of a healthy lifestyle. People are increasingly seeking effective ways to shed excess weight and reduce body fat. This pursuit often involves a combination of dietary changes, exercise, and lifestyle adjustments.

The Science Behind Weight Loss

Weight loss occurs when there is a calorie deficit, meaning you burn more calories than you consume. To achieve this, many individuals turn to various diets, such as low-carb, low-fat, or intermittent fasting. One popular approach is the ketogenic diet, which emphasizes high-fat and low-carb intake to induce a state of ketosis, where the body burns fat for energy.

Key Points to Consider:

- **Caloric Intake:** Reducing caloric intake is fundamental to weight loss. Cutting back on portion sizes and choosing nutrient-dense foods can help.

- **Exercise:** Combining a balanced diet with regular physical activity is essential for effective fat burning. Cardiovascular exercises like running and strength training can help boost metabolism.

- **Metabolism:** Metabolic rate varies among individuals. Some people have a naturally faster metabolism, while others may have a slower one. Understanding your metabolism can inform your weight loss strategy.

Effective Fat-Burning Foods

Certain foods are known for their fat-burning properties. Incorporating these into your diet can support your weight loss efforts.

1. Green Tea: Green tea contains compounds like catechins and caffeine that can boost metabolism and increase fat oxidation.

2. Lean Proteins: Foods like chicken, turkey, and tofu are high in protein and can help control appetite and build lean muscle.

3. Whole Grains: Whole grains like quinoa and oats provide sustained energy and can prevent overeating by keeping you full.

4. Spicy Foods: Spices like cayenne pepper contain capsaicin, which may increase metabolism and reduce appetite.

5. Nuts and Seeds: These are rich in healthy fats and can help you stay satiated throughout the day.

Challenges in Achieving Sustainable Weight Loss

Sustainable weight loss can be challenging due to various factors, including lifestyle, emotional eating, and metabolic differences. It's essential to set realistic goals and seek support when needed. Crash diets or extreme weight loss measures are often unsustainable and can lead to health problems.

Improved Energy Levels and Mental Clarity

Another compelling aspect of dietary choices is their impact on energy levels and mental clarity. The food we consume has a direct influence on our cognitive function and overall vitality.

The Role of Nutrient-Rich Foods

Eating a balanced diet rich in essential nutrients is crucial for maintaining high energy levels and mental clarity. Key nutrients include:

1. Omega-3 Fatty Acids: Found in fatty fish like salmon, omega-3s support brain health and can enhance cognitive function.

2. B Vitamins: B vitamins, such as B6 and B12, are essential for energy production and can help reduce fatigue.

3. Complex Carbohydrates: Whole grains and starchy vegetables provide a steady source of energy by regulating blood sugar levels.

4. Antioxidants: Fruits and vegetables rich in antioxidants combat oxidative stress and support brain health.

The Connection Between Diet and Brain Health

Dietary choices can impact mental clarity and cognitive function. For instance, a diet high in processed foods, sugar, and trans fats may lead to brain fog and reduced mental sharpness. In contrast, a diet rich in whole foods can improve focus and concentration.

Ketogenic Diet and Mental Clarity: Some individuals report improved mental clarity and focus when following a ketogenic diet, which is believed to be linked to stable blood sugar levels and the production of ketones in the brain.

Lifestyle Factors for Enhanced Mental Clarity

In addition to diet, lifestyle factors play a significant role in mental clarity and energy levels. These include:

- **Adequate Sleep:** Getting enough quality sleep is essential for cognitive function.

- **Stress Management:** Chronic stress can impair mental clarity, so stress-reduction techniques are valuable.

- **Regular Exercise:** Physical activity increases blood flow to the brain and promotes mental alertness.

Managing Health Conditions with the Diet

Diet plays a pivotal role in managing various health conditions. Whether it's diabetes, heart disease, or autoimmune disorders, the food we eat can either exacerbate or alleviate symptoms.

Diabetes Management

For individuals with diabetes, maintaining stable blood sugar levels is essential. This can be achieved through:

1. Carbohydrate Monitoring: Keeping track of carbohydrate intake and choosing complex carbs over simple sugars helps regulate blood sugar.

2. High-Fiber Foods: Fiber-rich foods like beans and whole grains can slow down the absorption of glucose.

3. Lean Proteins: Incorporating lean proteins into meals

can help stabilize blood sugar.

4. Portion Control: Monitoring portion sizes prevents blood sugar spikes.

Heart-Healthy Diet

A heart-healthy diet can reduce the risk of heart disease by:

1. Reducing Saturated Fat: Limiting saturated fat from sources like red meat and full-fat dairy products.

2. Increasing Omega-3s: Eating fatty fish, flaxseeds, and walnuts for heart-protective omega-3 fatty acids.

3. Lowering Sodium: Reducing salt intake to maintain healthy blood pressure.

Autoimmune Disorders

Certain autoimmune disorders, like celiac disease, require strict dietary adherence to manage symptoms. In the case of celiac disease, a gluten-free diet is necessary to prevent gastrointestinal discomfort and other health issues.

CHAPTER THREE

Getting Started

Preparing Mentally for the Carnivore Diet

The Carnivore Diet is a dietary approach that has gained popularity in recent years. It involves consuming exclusively animal products, primarily meat, and animal-derived foods while excluding all plant-based foods. Transitioning to such a restrictive diet can be mentally challenging, but with the right mindset and preparation, it can be a rewarding experience. Here's how to prepare mentally for the Carnivore Diet.

Understanding the Basics

Before embarking on the Carnivore Diet, it's essential to educate yourself about its fundamentals. Learn about the primary foods allowed on the diet, which include beef, pork, poultry, fish, and animal fats. Understand the philosophy behind it, which emphasizes the potential benefits of animal-based nutrition, such as improved energy levels, weight loss, and mental clarity.

Setting Clear Goals

Setting clear and achievable goals is crucial for success on the Carnivore Diet. Determine your reasons for choosing this diet, whether it's for health reasons, weight loss, or experimentation. Having well-defined goals will help you stay motivated and committed, even when faced with challenges.

Overcoming Mental Blocks

Many people have preconceived notions about a diet that excludes plant-based foods. It's essential to overcome these mental blocks and myths associated with the Carnivore Diet. Seek out reputable sources of information, consult with healthcare professionals, and connect with online communities of Carnivore Diet enthusiasts to gain insights and support.

Preparing for Detoxification

Transitioning to the Carnivore Diet may involve a period of detoxification as your body adapts to a new way of eating. Some individuals experience symptoms such as fatigue, headaches, and digestive changes during this phase. Mentally prepare for this by understanding that these symptoms are often temporary and a sign that your body is adjusting.

Embracing Variety within the Diet

While the Carnivore Diet may seem limited, there's still room for variety within the animal-based foods you can consume. Explore different cuts of meat, cooking methods, and seasoning options to keep your meals interesting and satisfying. Embracing this variety can help you stay mentally engaged with your diet.

Cultivating a Positive Mindset

Maintaining a positive mindset is essential when adopting any new dietary approach. Focus on the benefits you hope to achieve, such as improved health, increased energy, or weight loss. Practice mindfulness and self-compassion to navigate any challenges that may arise.

Creating a Meal Plan and Setting Goals

To succeed on the Carnivore Diet, it's crucial to have a well-structured meal plan and clear goals in place. Here's a step-by-step guide on how to create a meal plan and set achievable goals for this unique dietary approach.

Assess Your Current Diet

Before transitioning to the Carnivore Diet, take stock of your current eating habits. Identify the foods you'll need to eliminate and those you'll incorporate into your new plan. This assessment will serve as a starting point for your meal plan.

Define Your Nutritional Goals

Determine your nutritional goals for the Carnivore Diet. Are you primarily focused on weight loss, muscle gain, improved digestion, or overall health? Your goals will influence the composition of your meals and your calorie intake.

Plan Your Meals

Create a weekly meal plan that outlines what you'll eat for breakfast, lunch, dinner, and snacks. Since the Carnivore Diet is relatively restrictive, focus on incorporating a variety of animal products, such as beef, poultry, fish, and organ meats, to ensure you receive essential nutrients.

Calculate Macronutrients

To meet your nutritional goals, calculate the macronutrient ratios that work best for you. The Carnivore Diet typically emphasizes a high-fat, moderate-protein, and low-carbohydrate intake. Adjust these ratios based on your specific objectives.

Consider Supplements

While the Carnivore Diet can provide most essential nutrients, some individuals may benefit from supplements such as vitamin D, omega-3 fatty acids, and electrolytes. Consult with a healthcare professional to determine if supplements are necessary for your diet.

Monitor Progress

Regularly track your progress to ensure you're meeting your goals. Keep a food diary to record what you eat and how you feel. Adjust your meal plan as needed to optimize your results.

Stay Hydrated

Hydration is essential on any diet, including the Carnivore Diet. While you won't be consuming fruits and vegetables, be sure to drink an adequate amount of water to support overall health and digestion.

Seek Professional Guidance

If you're unsure about creating a meal plan or setting goals for the Carnivore Diet, consider consulting with a registered dietitian or nutritionist. They can provide personalized guidance and ensure you're meeting your nutritional needs.

Stocking Your Kitchen with Carnivore Diet Essentials

A well-stocked kitchen is the foundation for successfully following the Carnivore Diet. Since this diet primarily consists of animal products, it's essential to have the right essentials on hand to create delicious and nutritious meals. Here's a comprehensive guide to stocking your kitchen for the Carnivore Diet.

High-Quality Meats

Invest in high-quality meats, as they will be the

cornerstone of your Carnivore Diet. Opt for grass-fed beef, pasture-raised poultry, wild-caught fish, and organ meats whenever possible. These choices are not only more nutritious but also align with the diet's principles.

Animal Fats

Animal fats such as lard, tallow, and duck fat are essential for cooking and adding flavor to your meals. Keep these fats in your kitchen to use as cooking oils and to enhance the taste of your dishes.

Bone Broth

Bone broth is a nutrient-dense and flavorful addition to the Carnivore Diet. You can make your own by simmering animal bones or purchase pre-made bone broth from reputable sources. It can serve as a warming and nourishing beverage.

Salt and Seasonings

While the Carnivore Diet is simple in its food choices, you can still add flavor with high-quality salt and seasonings. Opt for natural sea salt or Himalayan salt, and consider using herbs and spices like black pepper, garlic powder, and rosemary to enhance your meals.

Cooking Equipment

Ensure you have the necessary cooking equipment, such as a grill, stovetop, oven, and cast-iron skillet. These tools will allow you to prepare a wide variety of carnivore-friendly dishes.

Storage Containers

Invest in quality storage containers to keep your meats and cooked dishes fresh. Proper storage is crucial for maintaining food safety and preventing waste.

Refrigeration

Make sure your refrigerator and freezer have enough space to store your meat and animal products. Consider investing in a separate freezer if you plan to buy meat in bulk.

Online Resources

Explore online resources and specialty stores that cater to Carnivore Diet enthusiasts. You can find unique products like grass-fed jerky, pemmican, and bone marrow supplements to enhance your diet.

Tips for Dining Out While on the Diet

Dining out while following the Carnivore Diet can be challenging, as many restaurants predominantly offer plant-based and carb-heavy options. However, with some strategic planning and communication, you can enjoy dining out while staying true to your dietary principles. Here are some helpful tips for navigating restaurants on the Carnivore Diet.

Research Restaurants in Advance

Before heading out to a restaurant, research the menu online or call ahead to inquire about their meat-centric options. Look for steakhouses, barbecue joints, and seafood restaurants that are more likely to have suitable choices.

Be Clear About Your Dietary Needs

When you arrive at the restaurant, don't hesitate to communicate your dietary needs to the server. Politely explain that you are following the Carnivore Diet and would like to order meat or animal-based dishes without any sauces, marinades, or sides.

Customize Your Order

Many restaurants are willing to accommodate special dietary requests. Customize your order by asking for a plain steak, grilled chicken, or a seafood dish without any added ingredients. Request that your food be cooked in animal fats like butter or lard.

Focus on the Protein

On the Carnivore Diet, your primary focus should be on getting enough protein. Choose protein-rich options like ribeye steak, salmon, or grilled chicken breast. Skip the starches and vegetables typically served as sides.

Avoid Sauces and Condiments

Be cautious about sauces, condiments, and dressings, as they often contain hidden sugars and additives. Request that these items be omitted from your meal, or ask for olive oil and vinegar for a simple dressing.

Embrace Water and Black Coffee

While many people enjoy pairing their meals with alcoholic beverages or sugary drinks, stick to water or black coffee when dining out. These options are Carnivore Diet-friendly and won't derail your dietary efforts.

Practice Portion Control

Restaurant portions are often larger than what you might typically eat at home. Practice portion control by eating until you are satisfied and requesting a to-go container for leftovers.

Dessert Alternatives

If you have a sweet tooth, consider alternatives like a cheese plate or a small serving of plain yogurt for dessert.

These options can satisfy cravings while staying within the Carnivore Diet guidelines.

Don't Stress Over Occasional Deviations

It's important to remember that occasional deviations from the Carnivore Diet, especially when dining out, are normal and shouldn't cause undue stress. Focus on making the best choices available to you in each situation.

CHAPTER FOUR

Carnivore Diet Recipes

Section 1: Breakfast

Steak and Eggs

Description of the Meal: Steak and eggs is a classic breakfast dish that combines the rich, savory flavors of steak with the protein-packed goodness of eggs. It's a hearty and satisfying meal that will keep you energized throughout the day.

Ingredients:

- 2 sirloin steaks (6-8 oz each)
- 4 large eggs
- 2 tablespoons olive oil
- Salt and pepper, to taste
- Fresh parsley, for garnish (optional)

Instructions:

1. Start by seasoning the sirloin steaks with salt and pepper on both sides. Let them sit at room temperature for about 15 minutes to allow the flavors to meld.

2. Heat a skillet or frying pan over medium-high heat and add the olive oil. When the oil is hot, add the steaks and cook to your desired level

of doneness, about 3-4 minutes per side for medium-rare. Adjust the cooking time based on your preference.

3. While the steaks are cooking, prepare the eggs. You can either scramble them or cook them sunny-side-up or over-easy, depending on your preference.

4. Once the steaks are done, remove them from the pan and let them rest for a few minutes before slicing.

5. Plate the sliced steak alongside the eggs. Garnish with fresh parsley if desired.

6. Enjoy your delicious steak and eggs breakfast!

Nutritional Information: (Per Serving)

- Calories: 450
- Protein: 42g
- Fat: 30g
- Carbohydrates: 2g
- Fiber: 0g

Bacon and Avocado Scramble

Description of the Meal: Bacon and avocado scramble is a flavorful and satisfying breakfast option that combines crispy bacon with creamy avocado and fluffy scrambled eggs. It's a perfect blend of textures and tastes to kickstart your day.

Ingredients:

- 4 slices of bacon, chopped
- 4 large eggs
- 1 ripe avocado, diced

- Salt and pepper, to taste
- Fresh chives, for garnish (optional)

Instructions:

1. In a skillet, cook the chopped bacon over medium heat until it becomes crispy. Remove the bacon from the skillet and drain excess fat on paper towels.

2. In a bowl, beat the eggs and season them with salt and pepper.

3. Pour the beaten eggs into the same skillet and cook over medium-low heat, stirring gently, until they are just set.

4. Add the diced avocado to the scrambled eggs and continue to cook for another minute, allowing the avocado to warm through.

5. Sprinkle the crispy bacon pieces over the top of the scramble.

6. Garnish with fresh chives if desired.

7. Serve the bacon and avocado scramble hot.

Nutritional Information: (Per Serving)

- Calories: 320
- Protein: 16g
- Fat: 25g
- Carbohydrates: 6g
- Fiber: 4g

Sausage Patties with Cheese

Description of the Meal: Sausage patties with cheese are a savory and cheesy breakfast delight. These homemade sausage patties are packed with flavor and are perfect for those who enjoy a hearty start to their day.

Ingredients:

- 1 lb ground pork sausage
- 1/2 cup shredded cheddar cheese
- 1/4 cup breadcrumbs
- 1/4 cup finely chopped onion
- 1/2 teaspoon garlic powder
- Salt and pepper, to taste

Instructions:

1. In a mixing bowl, combine the ground pork sausage, shredded cheddar cheese, breadcrumbs, chopped onion, garlic powder, salt, and pepper. Mix until all the ingredients are well incorporated.

2. Divide the mixture into equal portions and shape them into patties.

3. Heat a skillet over medium-high heat and add a bit of oil if needed. Place the sausage patties in the skillet and cook for about 4-5 minutes on each side, or until they are browned and cooked through.

4. Remove the sausage patties from the skillet and drain any excess fat on paper towels.

5. Serve the sausage patties hot with your favorite breakfast sides.

Nutritional Information: (Per Serving)

- Calories: 380
- Protein: 18g
- Fat: 30g

- Carbohydrates: 6g
- Fiber: 1g

Coffee with Butter and Coconut Oil

Description of the Meal: Coffee with butter and coconut oil, also known as "bulletproof coffee," is a creamy and frothy beverage that provides a burst of energy. It's a popular choice for those following a ketogenic or low-carb diet.

Ingredients:

- 1 cup brewed coffee
- 1 tablespoon unsalted butter
- 1 tablespoon coconut oil

Instructions:

1. Brew a cup of your favorite coffee using your preferred method.

2. In a blender, combine the hot coffee, unsalted butter, and coconut oil.

3. Blend on high speed for about 20-30 seconds until the coffee is frothy and the fats are well incorporated.

4. Pour the bulletproof coffee into a mug and enjoy while hot.

Nutritional Information: (Per Serving)

- Calories: 210
- Protein: 0g
- Fat: 24g
- Carbohydrates: 0g
- Fiber: 0g

Section 2: Lunch

Ribeye Steak Salad

Description of the Meal: Ribeye Steak Salad is a delightful combination of tender, grilled ribeye steak slices served on a bed of fresh greens and vibrant vegetables. This salad is perfect for those seeking a hearty and protein-packed meal with a burst of flavors.

Ingredients:

- 1 ribeye steak (8-10 ounces)
- 4 cups mixed greens (lettuce, spinach, arugula)
- 1/2 cup cherry tomatoes, halved
- 1/4 red onion, thinly sliced
- 1/4 cup crumbled blue cheese
- 2 tablespoons balsamic vinaigrette dressing
- Salt and black pepper to taste
- Olive oil for grilling

Instructions:

1. Preheat your grill to medium-high heat. Brush the ribeye steak with a little olive oil and season generously with salt and black pepper.

2. Place the seasoned steak on the grill and cook for about 4-5 minutes on each side for medium-rare doneness. Adjust the cooking time to your desired level of doneness.

3. Remove the steak from the grill and let it rest for 5 minutes to allow the juices to redistribute. Then, thinly slice it against the grain.

4. In a large salad bowl, combine the mixed greens, cherry tomatoes, red onion, and crumbled blue

cheese.

5. Drizzle the balsamic vinaigrette dressing over the salad and toss gently to coat.

6. Arrange the sliced ribeye steak on top of the salad.

7. Serve immediately, and enjoy this delicious Ribeye Steak Salad!

Nutritional Information:

- Calories: 450
- Protein: 35g
- Carbohydrates: 8g
- Fat: 30g
- Fiber: 2g

Salmon with Lemon Butter

Description of the Meal: Salmon with Lemon Butter is a classic seafood dish that combines the rich, buttery flavor of salmon with the zesty brightness of lemon. This recipe results in tender and flaky salmon fillets that are perfect for a healthy and flavorful meal.

Ingredients:

- 2 salmon fillets (6-8 ounces each)
- 2 tablespoons unsalted butter
- 2 cloves garlic, minced
- Juice of 1 lemon
- Zest of 1 lemon
- Salt and black pepper to taste
- Fresh parsley for garnish

Instructions:

1. Preheat your oven to 375°F (190°C).

2. In a small saucepan over medium heat, melt the butter. Add minced garlic and sauté for 1-2 minutes until fragrant but not browned.

3. Stir in the lemon juice and lemon zest. Remove from heat.

4. Season the salmon fillets with salt and black pepper on both sides.

5. Place the salmon fillets in an oven-safe baking dish.

6. Pour the lemon butter mixture over the salmon.

7. Bake in the preheated oven for 15-20 minutes or until the salmon easily flakes with a fork.

8. Garnish with fresh parsley and serve hot with your choice of side dishes.

Nutritional Information:

- Calories: 320
- Protein: 30g
- Carbohydrates: 2g
- Fat: 21g
- Fiber: 0.5g

Ground Beef Lettuce Wraps

Description of the Meal: Ground Beef Lettuce Wraps are a low-carb and satisfying meal option. These wraps are packed with seasoned ground beef and an assortment of fresh toppings, making them a flavorful and healthy choice.

Ingredients:

- 1 pound ground beef

- 1 tablespoon olive oil
- 1 small onion, finely chopped
- 2 cloves garlic, minced
- 1 red bell pepper, diced
- 1 zucchini, diced
- 1 teaspoon chili powder
- 1 teaspoon cumin
- Salt and black pepper to taste
- Iceberg lettuce leaves, for wrapping
- Toppings: diced tomatoes, avocado slices, shredded cheese, sour cream, and salsa

Instructions:

1. In a large skillet, heat olive oil over medium heat. Add chopped onion and garlic and sauté until translucent.

2. Add ground beef to the skillet and cook until browned, breaking it into crumbles with a spatula.

3. Stir in diced red bell pepper and zucchini. Cook for an additional 3-4 minutes until the vegetables soften.

4. Season the mixture with chili powder, cumin, salt, and black pepper. Mix well.

5. Wash and separate iceberg lettuce leaves, creating cups for the filling.

6. Spoon the ground beef mixture into the lettuce cups.

7. Add your choice of toppings, such as diced

tomatoes, avocado slices, shredded cheese, sour cream, and salsa.

8. Serve the Ground Beef Lettuce Wraps immediately for a tasty and carb-friendly meal.

Nutritional Information:

- Calories: 320
- Protein: 25g
- Carbohydrates: 7g
- Fat: 21g
- Fiber: 2g

Chicken Thigh Skewers

Description of the Meal: Chicken Thigh Skewers are a savory and succulent dish that combines marinated chicken thighs with flavorful herbs and spices. These skewers are perfect for grilling and make for a delicious appetizer or main course.

Ingredients:

- 8 boneless, skinless chicken thighs
- 1/4 cup olive oil
- 2 cloves garlic, minced
- 1 tablespoon lemon juice
- 1 teaspoon paprika
- 1 teaspoon dried oregano
- Salt and black pepper to taste
- Wooden skewers, soaked in water
- Fresh parsley for garnish

Instructions:

1. In a bowl, whisk together olive oil, minced garlic,

lemon juice, paprika, dried oregano, salt, and black pepper to create the marinade.

2. Cut the chicken thighs into bite-sized pieces and place them in a resealable plastic bag or a shallow dish.

3. Pour the marinade over the chicken and toss to coat evenly. Seal the bag or cover the dish and refrigerate for at least 30 minutes, or ideally, marinate for 2-4 hours.

4. Preheat your grill to medium-high heat.

5. Thread the marinated chicken pieces onto the soaked wooden skewers.

6. Grill the chicken skewers for about 6-8 minutes per side, or until they are cooked through and have nice grill marks.

7. Garnish with fresh parsley and serve hot with your favorite dipping sauce.

Nutritional Information:

- Calories: 280
- Protein: 30g
- Carbohydrates: 2g
- Fat: 16g
- Fiber: 0.5g

Section 3: Dinner

T-bone steak with garlic butter

Description of the Meal: Treat yourself to a classic and indulgent T-bone steak with garlic butter. This dish combines the rich flavors of a perfectly cooked steak with the creamy goodness of garlic butter.

Ingredients:

- 1 T-bone steak (about 1 pound)
- 2 cloves garlic, minced
- 2 tablespoons unsalted butter
- Salt and black pepper, to taste
- Fresh parsley, chopped for garnish

Instructions:

1. Preheat your grill or stovetop skillet over high heat. Make sure it's very hot for that perfect sear.

2. Season the T-bone steak generously with salt and black pepper on both sides.

3. Place the steak on the hot grill or skillet and cook for about 4-5 minutes on each side for medium-rare. Adjust the cooking time based on your desired level of doneness.

4. While the steak is cooking, prepare the garlic butter. In a small saucepan, melt the butter over low heat. Add the minced garlic and sauté for about 1-2 minutes until fragrant. Remove from heat.

5. Once the steak is done, transfer it to a plate and let it rest for a few minutes.

6. Pour the garlic butter over the rested T-bone steak, allowing it to melt and coat the meat.

7. Garnish with fresh chopped parsley.

8. Slice the T-bone steak against the grain and serve hot with your choice of side dishes.

Nutritional Information:

- Calories: 550

- Protein: 40g
- Carbohydrates: 1g
- Fat: 42g
- Fiber: 0g

Pork chops with herbs

Description of the Meal: Pork chops with herbs is a flavorful and aromatic dish that combines tender pork chops with a medley of herbs and spices for a delightful meal.

Ingredients:

- 4 bone-in pork chops
- 2 tablespoons olive oil
- 2 cloves garlic, minced
- 1 teaspoon dried thyme
- 1 teaspoon dried rosemary
- Salt and black pepper, to taste
- Fresh parsley, chopped for garnish

Instructions:

1. Preheat your oven to 375°F (190°C).
2. Season the pork chops with salt and black pepper on both sides.
3. In an ovenproof skillet, heat the olive oil over medium-high heat. Add the minced garlic and sauté for about 1 minute until fragrant.
4. Add the pork chops to the skillet and sear for 2-3 minutes on each side until they develop a golden brown crust.

5. Sprinkle dried thyme and rosemary evenly over the pork chops.

6. Transfer the skillet to the preheated oven and bake for 15-20 minutes or until the pork chops reach an internal temperature of 145°F (63°C).

7. Remove from the oven and let the pork chops rest for a few minutes.

8. Garnish with fresh chopped parsley and serve hot with your choice of sides.

Nutritional Information:

- Calories: 320
- Protein: 30g
- Carbohydrates: 1g
- Fat: 22g
- Fiber: 0g

Lamb chops with mint sauce

Description of the Meal: Lamb chops with mint sauce is a classic combination that brings out the tender and succulent flavors of lamb paired with the freshness of mint.

Ingredients:

- 8 lamb chops
- 2 tablespoons olive oil
- 2 cloves garlic, minced
- 1/4 cup fresh mint leaves, chopped
- 2 tablespoons red wine vinegar
- Salt and black pepper, to taste

Instructions:

1. Preheat your grill to medium-high heat.

2. Season the lamb chops with salt and black pepper on both sides.

3. In a small bowl, mix together the minced garlic, chopped mint leaves, olive oil, and red wine vinegar to create the mint sauce.

4. Grill the lamb chops for about 3-4 minutes on each side for medium-rare or adjust the cooking time according to your preference.

5. Once done, remove the lamb chops from the grill and let them rest for a few minutes.

6. Serve the lamb chops hot, drizzled with the mint sauce.

Nutritional Information:

- Calories: 380
- Protein: 36g
- Carbohydrates: 1g
- Fat: 26g
- Fiber: 0g

Bison burger with cheese

Description of the Meal: Indulge in a juicy bison burger with cheese, a lean and flavorful alternative to traditional beef burgers that's topped with melted cheese.

Ingredients:

- 1 bison burger patty (about 1/3 pound)

- 1 hamburger bun
- 1 slice of your favorite cheese
- Lettuce, tomato, onion (optional toppings)
- Ketchup and mustard (optional condiments)

Instructions:

1. Preheat your grill or stovetop skillet over medium-high heat.

2. Season the bison burger patty with salt and black pepper on both sides.

3. Place the burger patty on the hot grill or skillet and cook for about 3-4 minutes on each side for medium-rare, or adjust the cooking time to your desired level of doneness.

4. During the last minute of cooking, place the cheese slice on top of the burger patty to melt.

5. Toast the hamburger bun on the grill or in a toaster until it's lightly browned.

6. Assemble your bison burger by placing the cooked patty on the bottom bun. Add lettuce, tomato, onion, ketchup, and mustard if desired. Top with the other half of the bun.

7. Serve hot with your favorite side dishes.

Nutritional Information:

- Calories: 400
- Protein: 35g
- Carbohydrates: 25g
- Fat: 18g
- Fiber: 2g

Section 4: Snacks and Side Dishes

Beef Jerky

Description of the Meal: Beef jerky is a savory and protein-packed snack made from thinly sliced beef that's been marinated and dried. It's a perfect on-the-go option for a quick energy boost.

Ingredients:

- 1 pound of lean beef (such as sirloin or flank steak)
- 1/4 cup soy sauce
- 2 tablespoons Worcestershire sauce
- 2 teaspoons smoked paprika
- 1 teaspoon garlic powder
- 1 teaspoon onion powder
- 1/2 teaspoon black pepper
- 1/2 teaspoon red pepper flakes (adjust for spice level)
- 1 tablespoon brown sugar (optional, for sweetness)

Instructions:

1. **Preparation:** Start by freezing the beef for about 30 minutes to make it easier to slice thinly. Slice the partially frozen beef into 1/8-inch thick strips, removing any visible fat.

2. **Marinating:** In a bowl, combine soy sauce, Worcestershire sauce, smoked paprika, garlic powder, onion powder, black pepper, red pepper flakes, and brown sugar if you prefer a touch of sweetness. Place the sliced beef in a resealable plastic bag and pour the marinade over it. Seal the bag, removing as much air as possible, and

massage the marinade into the beef. Marinate in the refrigerator for at least 4 hours or overnight.

3. **Dehydrating:** Preheat your oven to the lowest possible setting (usually around 170°F or 75°C). Place the marinated beef strips on a wire rack set on a baking sheet. Make sure they are not touching. You can also use a food dehydrator if you have one. Bake or dehydrate for 4-6 hours until the beef jerky is dry, but still pliable.

4. **Cooling:** Let the beef jerky cool to room temperature. Pat it dry with paper towels to remove any excess moisture.

5. **Storage:** Store the beef jerky in an airtight container or resealable bags. It can be kept at room temperature for a few days or in the refrigerator for longer shelf life.

Nutritional Information:

- Serving Size: 1 ounce (about 28g)
- Calories: 70
- Protein: 10g
- Fat: 2g
- Carbohydrates: 2g
- Fiber: 0g

Deviled Eggs

Description of the Meal: Deviled eggs are a classic appetizer or snack made from hard-boiled eggs filled with a creamy and flavorful yolk mixture. They're a crowd-pleasing favorite at parties and gatherings.

Ingredients:

- 6 large eggs
- 2 tablespoons mayonnaise
- 1 teaspoon Dijon mustard
- 1/2 teaspoon white vinegar
- Salt and pepper to taste
- Paprika for garnish
- Chopped fresh chives for garnish (optional)

Instructions:

1. **Boiling Eggs:** Place the eggs in a saucepan and cover them with cold water. Bring the water to a boil over high heat. Once boiling, reduce the heat to low and simmer for 9-12 minutes.

2. **Cooling and Peeling:** Drain the hot water and transfer the eggs to a bowl of ice water to cool for about 5 minutes. Gently tap each egg on a hard surface to crack the shell, then peel them.

3. **Cutting and Filling:** Cut the eggs in half lengthwise. Carefully remove the yolks and place them in a bowl. Mash the yolks with a fork and add mayonnaise, Dijon mustard, white vinegar, salt, and pepper. Mix until smooth.

4. **Filling the Eggs:** Spoon the yolk mixture back into the egg white halves or use a piping bag for a decorative touch.

5. **Garnishing:** Sprinkle paprika on top for flavor and color. You can also garnish with chopped fresh chives if desired.

6. **Chilling:** Refrigerate the deviled eggs for at least 30 minutes before serving.

Nutritional Information:

- Serving Size: 2 halves
- Calories: 100
- Protein: 6g
- Fat: 8g
- Carbohydrates: 1g
- Fiber: 0g

Zucchini Noodles with Meat Sauce

Description of the Meal: Zucchini noodles with meat sauce is a low-carb and healthy alternative to traditional pasta. It's a satisfying dish that combines the flavors of a rich meat sauce with tender zucchini noodles.

Ingredients:

- 2 large zucchinis
- 1 pound lean ground beef or turkey
- 1 onion, finely chopped
- 2 cloves garlic, minced
- 1 can (14 ounces) crushed tomatoes
- 1 teaspoon dried basil
- 1 teaspoon dried oregano
- Salt and pepper to taste
- Grated Parmesan cheese for garnish (optional)

Instructions:

1. **Preparing Zucchini Noodles:** Use a spiralizer or a julienne peeler to create zucchini noodles (zoodles). Set them aside on paper towels to absorb excess moisture.

2. **Cooking Meat Sauce:** In a large skillet, brown

the ground beef or turkey over medium heat, breaking it into crumbles as it cooks. Drain any excess fat. Add chopped onion and garlic, and sauté until they become translucent.

3. **Adding Tomatoes and Spices:** Pour in the crushed tomatoes, dried basil, dried oregano, salt, and pepper. Stir well and let the sauce simmer for about 10-15 minutes to develop flavor.

4. **Cooking Zucchini Noodles:** While the sauce simmers, heat a separate skillet over medium heat. Add the zucchini noodles and sauté for 2-3 minutes until they are just tender. Avoid overcooking to maintain their texture.

5. **Serving:** Serve the zucchini noodles with the meat sauce on top. Garnish with grated Parmesan cheese if desired.

Nutritional Information:

- Serving Size: 1/4 of the recipe
- Calories: 275
- Protein: 26g
- Fat: 15g
- Carbohydrates: 10g
- Fiber: 3g

Creamed Spinach

Description of the Meal: Creamed spinach is a rich and creamy side dish made with tender spinach leaves in a velvety sauce. It's a comforting and nutritious addition to any meal.

Ingredients:

- 1 pound fresh spinach leaves, washed and stemmed
- 2 tablespoons butter
- 2 cloves garlic, minced
- 1/4 cup heavy cream
- 1/4 cup grated Parmesan cheese
- Salt and pepper to taste
- Pinch of nutmeg (optional)

Instructions:

1. **Blanching the Spinach:** Bring a large pot of salted water to a boil. Add the spinach and blanch for about 1-2 minutes until wilted. Drain the spinach and immediately transfer it to a bowl of ice water to stop the cooking process. Squeeze out excess water and chop the spinach.

2. **Making the Sauce:** In a large skillet, melt the butter over medium heat. Add minced garlic and sauté for about 1 minute until fragrant.

3. **Creamy Mixture:** Stir in the heavy cream and grated Parmesan cheese. Cook, stirring constantly, until the mixture thickens and the cheese is melted.

4. **Adding Spinach:** Add the chopped spinach to the creamy sauce. Season with salt, pepper, and a pinch of nutmeg if desired. Cook for another 2-3 minutes until the spinach is heated through.

5. **Serving:** Serve the creamed spinach as a side dish alongside your favorite main course.

Nutritional Information:

- Serving Size: 1/4 of the recipe

- Calories: 180
- Protein: 6g
- Fat: 15g
- Carbohydrates: 6g
- Fiber: 2g

CHAPTER FIVE

Carnivore Diet Success Tips

Staying consistent and committed

Consistency and commitment are key factors in achieving any goal, whether it's related to your health, career, or personal life. When it comes to staying consistent and committed, it's essential to understand the psychology behind it and employ effective strategies.

Understanding the Importance of Consistency Consistency is the backbone of success. It's about doing something repeatedly over time, which builds momentum and leads to progress. Think of consistency as the steady drip of water that eventually forms a deep well. Without it, your efforts might fizzle out, leaving you frustrated and disheartened.

Setting Clear Goals To stay consistent, you need clear, well-defined goals. These goals act as your compass, guiding your actions and decisions. Without a destination in mind, it's easy to lose motivation. When setting goals, make them specific, measurable, achievable, relevant, and time-bound (SMART). This clarity will help you stay committed.

Creating a Routine Routines provide structure and make it easier to stay on track. They eliminate the need to make decisions constantly, reducing decision fatigue. Whether it's waking up early to exercise, setting aside time for work or study, or allocating moments for self-care, a routine helps you form positive habits.

Building Accountability Accountability can be a powerful motivator. Share your goals with a friend, family member, or mentor who can hold you responsible for your progress. Consider joining a group or community that shares similar objectives. Knowing that others are watching can encourage you to stay consistent.

Handling Setbacks Consistency doesn't mean perfection. You will encounter setbacks along the way. The key is not to let these setbacks derail your commitment. Instead, view them as learning opportunities. Analyze what went wrong, make necessary adjustments, and keep moving forward.

Rewards and Celebrations Celebrate your achievements, no matter how small they may seem. Rewards provide positive reinforcement and can boost your commitment. Treat yourself when you reach milestones—it could be a spa day, a favorite meal, or simply acknowledging your progress.

Dealing with cravings and temptation

Cravings and temptations are natural obstacles that can hinder your progress when trying to achieve a goal, especially when it comes to maintaining a healthy lifestyle. Learning to manage and overcome these cravings is essential for long-term success.

Understanding Cravings Cravings often arise from a combination of physiological, psychological, and environmental factors. It's crucial to recognize that cravings are a normal part of human experience. They are not a sign of weakness but rather a natural response to certain triggers.

Mindful Eating Practicing mindful eating can help you become more aware of your cravings and eating habits. Pay attention to physical hunger cues, and differentiate them from emotional triggers. By slowing down and savoring each bite, you can reduce the urge to give in to unhealthy temptations.

Healthy Alternatives Instead of succumbing to unhealthy temptations, explore healthier alternatives. If you're craving something sweet, opt for fresh fruits or dark chocolate. When craving salty snacks, try roasted nuts or air-popped popcorn. Finding nutritious substitutes can satisfy your cravings without derailing your progress.

Distraction Techniques When a craving strikes, distract yourself with a different activity. Engage in a hobby, go for a walk, call a friend, or read a book. Redirecting your focus away from the temptation can help weaken its grip on you.

Moderation and Planning Allow yourself to indulge occasionally, but do so in moderation. Depriving yourself completely may lead to intense cravings and binging later on. Plan your indulgences as part of your overall strategy to maintain control.

Seeking Support Don't be afraid to seek support from friends, family, or a therapist if you find it challenging to manage cravings on your own. Talking about your struggles can provide valuable insights and encouragement.

Tracking progress and making adjustments

Tracking your progress is vital to achieving any goal. It allows you to assess how far you've come and identify areas that may require adjustments. Here's how to effectively track your progress and make necessary changes along the way.

Setting Metrics Determine the specific metrics that align with your goal. For example, if your goal is fitness-related, track metrics like weight, body measurements, or workout performance. If it's a career goal, track metrics related to your performance, such as completed projects or revenue generated.

Consistent Measurement Regularly measure your chosen metrics to ensure consistency. Depending on your goal, this could be daily, weekly, or monthly. Consistency in measurement helps you identify trends and patterns over time.

Recording Data Keep a record of your progress. Use a journal, spreadsheet, or a goal-tracking app to log your measurements and observations. Having a historical record enables you to analyze your journey.

Review and Analysis Periodically review your progress data. Look for trends and patterns. Are you making steady progress, or have there been plateaus or setbacks? Analyzing this information helps you understand what's working and what needs adjustment.

Making Informed Adjustments Based on your analysis, make informed adjustments to your approach. If you've hit a plateau in your fitness journey, consider changing your workout routine or adjusting your diet. In your career, if you're not meeting your project deadlines, assess your time management strategies and make improvements.

Setting New Goals As you achieve your initial goals, set new ones that build upon your progress. This keeps you motivated and continually striving for improvement. Each new goal should be a logical next step in your journey.

Seeking Feedback Don't hesitate to seek feedback from mentors, coaches, or peers. They can offer valuable insights and suggestions for improvement that you may not have considered.

Incorporating exercise into your routine

Incorporating exercise into your daily routine is a cornerstone of a healthy lifestyle. It's not just about getting in shape; it's also about boosting your overall well-being and energy levels. Here's how to make exercise a consistent part of your life.

Choosing an Enjoyable Activity The first step to incorporating exercise is to choose an activity you genuinely enjoy. Whether it's dancing, swimming, hiking, or playing a sport, doing something you love makes it easier to stay committed.

Start Slowly and Progress Gradually If you're new to exercise or getting back into it after a break, start slowly. Don't overwhelm yourself with intense workouts right away. Gradually increase the intensity and duration as your fitness level improves.

Set Realistic Goals Set achievable fitness goals. This could be completing a 5K run, doing a certain number of push-ups, or reaching a specific weightlifting target. Realistic goals give you something to work toward and track your progress.

Create a Schedule Block out time in your daily or weekly schedule for exercise. Treat it as an important appointment that you can't miss. Consistency is key, so stick to your exercise routine as closely as possible.

Mix It Up Variety can keep your workouts interesting. Incorporate a mix of aerobic, strength, and flexibility exercises. Trying different activities also prevents boredom and plateaus.

Find an Exercise Buddy Exercising with a friend or partner can provide motivation and accountability. You're more likely to stick to your routine if you have someone to share it with.

Overcome Excuses Excuses can derail your exercise routine. Identify common excuses you use to skip workouts and challenge them. Lack of time can be overcome by shorter, more intense workouts, for example.

Prioritize Recovery Don't forget the importance of rest and recovery. Your body needs time to heal and adapt to exercise. Incorporate rest days into your routine to prevent burnout and reduce the risk of injury.

CHAPTER 6

Frequently Asked Questions

Addressing Common Concerns about the Carnivore Diet

The Carnivore Diet has gained considerable attention in recent years, with proponents claiming various health benefits. However, like any diet, it has also faced its fair share of criticism and concerns. In this comprehensive guide, we will address some of the common concerns associated with the Carnivore Diet and provide expert answers and advice to help you make an informed decision about whether this dietary approach is right for you.

1. Lack of Dietary Variety

Concern: One of the most frequent criticisms of the Carnivore Diet is its extreme lack of dietary variety. Critics argue that excluding most food groups, such as fruits, vegetables, and grains, can lead to nutritional deficiencies.

Expert Answer: While it's true that the Carnivore Diet is highly restrictive, it's important to note that proponents believe animal-based foods are nutritionally dense and provide all essential nutrients. They argue that early humans survived and thrived on meat-based diets. However, to mitigate the risk of nutrient deficiencies, it's essential to consume a wide variety of animal products, including red meat, poultry, fish, and organ meats.

Additionally, some carnivore dieters incorporate dairy products like cheese and butter for additional nutrients.

2. Fiber Intake

Concern: Critics argue that the Carnivore Diet's lack of fiber could lead to digestive issues, constipation, and an unhealthy gut microbiome.

Expert Answer: Fiber is indeed absent from the Carnivore Diet since it excludes plant-based foods. However, proponents claim that fiber may not be as essential as traditionally believed. They argue that high-fiber diets can sometimes lead to digestive discomfort and that the body can adapt to lower fiber intake over time. Some individuals even report improved digestion on the Carnivore Diet, but it's essential to monitor your own body's response and adjust accordingly.

3. Nutrient Deficiency

Concern: Critics worry that the Carnivore Diet might result in nutrient deficiencies, particularly in vitamins and minerals like vitamin C and potassium, which are commonly found in fruits and vegetables.

Expert Answer: While fruits and vegetables are excellent sources of many nutrients, carnivore dieters argue that animal products contain most, if not all, essential nutrients in sufficient quantities. For example, vitamin C can be obtained from organ meats and small amounts of fruits like berries, which are allowed on some versions of the Carnivore Diet. Additionally, they assert that animal foods provide highly bioavailable forms of nutrients that are more easily absorbed by the body.

4. Increased Risk of Heart Disease

Concern: Some critics express concerns about the potential link between the high consumption of saturated fats in the Carnivore Diet and an increased risk of heart disease.

Expert Answer: The association between saturated fat and heart disease has been debated for decades. While animal fats do contain saturated fats, proponents of the Carnivore Diet argue that the latest research challenges the conventional wisdom on dietary fat. They claim that many people on this diet experience improvements in cholesterol profiles, with increased levels of "good" HDL cholesterol and reduced levels of triglycerides. However, individual responses to dietary fat can vary, so it's crucial to monitor your cholesterol levels and consult with a healthcare professional.

5. Long-term Sustainability

Concern: Critics question the long-term sustainability of the Carnivore Diet, wondering if it's realistic to exclude most food groups for an extended period.

Expert Answer: The long-term sustainability of the Carnivore Diet is a valid concern. While some individuals have followed this diet for years without apparent issues, it can be challenging to maintain in the long run. To address this concern, many carnivore dieters advocate for a "flexible" approach, allowing occasional inclusion of non-carnivorous foods. Ultimately, the sustainability of the diet will depend on individual preferences and goals.

6. Impact on the Environment

Concern: Critics argue that the Carnivore Diet's emphasis on animal products can have a detrimental impact on the environment, contributing to deforestation and greenhouse gas emissions.

Expert Answer: It's undeniable that the production of animal products can have environmental consequences. Proponents of the Carnivore Diet, however, emphasize the importance of sourcing meat and other animal products from sustainable and regenerative agriculture practices. They believe that ethical and environmentally conscious choices can mitigate the diet's impact on the planet. Additionally, some argue that the overall reduction in food waste, as carnivore diets tend to be less reliant on processed foods, can be seen as an environmental benefit.

7. Lack of Long-term Research

Concern: Critics highlight the limited scientific research on the long-term effects of the Carnivore Diet, making it difficult to assess its safety and efficacy.

Expert Answer: It's true that there is a shortage of long-term studies specifically focused on the Carnivore Diet. However, proponents argue that this diet shares some similarities with other low-carb, high-fat diets, such as the ketogenic diet, which have been researched more extensively. While more research is needed, anecdotal evidence and short-term studies suggest potential benefits in terms of weight loss, improved metabolic health, and reduced inflammation. If you're considering the Carnivore Diet, it's crucial to monitor your health markers and consult with a healthcare provider regularly.

CONCLUSION

The Carnivore Diet: A Recap of Weight Loss Benefits

The Carnivore Diet has gained significant attention in recent years for its potential benefits, especially in the realm of weight loss. This unconventional approach to nutrition centers around the consumption of animal-based foods exclusively, omitting plant-based foods entirely. While it may seem counterintuitive, the Carnivore Diet has garnered a dedicated following and numerous success stories. In this discussion, we will delve into a recap of the benefits associated with the Carnivore Diet for weight loss.

1. Rapid Weight Loss

One of the most striking aspects of the Carnivore Diet is its ability to induce rapid weight loss. By eliminating carbohydrates and plant-based foods, the body enters a state of ketosis, where it primarily burns fat for energy. This metabolic shift leads to quick reductions in body fat, making it an attractive option for those looking to shed excess pounds efficiently.

2. Enhanced Satiety

One of the common challenges people face when attempting to lose weight is dealing with persistent feelings of hunger. The Carnivore Diet can be particularly helpful in this regard. Animal-based foods are rich in proteins and fats, which are highly satiating. This means that individuals on this diet often experience reduced cravings and a greater sense of fullness, making it easier to adhere to a calorie deficit.

3. Improved Insulin Sensitivity

Insulin sensitivity plays a crucial role in weight management. The Carnivore Diet has been shown to enhance insulin sensitivity, which means the body can more effectively regulate blood sugar levels. This can be particularly beneficial for individuals who struggle with insulin resistance, a common issue in obesity.

4. Elimination of Inflammatory Foods

The diet's exclusive focus on animal products eliminates many potentially inflammatory foods, such as grains, legumes, and certain vegetables. Inflammation can contribute to weight gain and hinder weight loss efforts. By avoiding these triggers, individuals on the Carnivore Diet may experience a reduction in overall inflammation.

5. Simplicity and Compliance

The Carnivore Diet's simplicity can be a major advantage for those seeking to lose weight. Unlike complex diets that require meticulous tracking of macros and meal planning, this diet involves straightforward food choices. This simplicity often translates to better compliance, as individuals find it easier to stick to a diet with fewer restrictions and calculations.

6. Enhanced Mental Clarity and Focus

While weight loss is often the primary goal, many Carnivore Diet enthusiasts report improved mental clarity and focus as an unexpected benefit. The steady supply of energy from fat metabolism may lead to enhanced cognitive function, making it easier to stay on track with dietary goals.

7. Reduction in Cravings

Carbohydrates, especially refined sugars, are notorious for triggering cravings. By eliminating these from the diet, individuals on the Carnivore Diet often experience a significant reduction in sugar cravings. This can be a game-changer for those trying to break free from unhealthy eating patterns.

In summary, the Carnivore Diet offers a unique approach to weight loss, characterized by rapid results, enhanced satiety, improved insulin sensitivity, the elimination of inflammatory foods, simplicity, mental clarity, and reduced cravings. However, it's essential to approach this diet with caution and consult with a healthcare professional, as it is highly restrictive and may not be suitable for everyone. As with any diet, individual results may vary, and it's crucial to prioritize long-term health and sustainability.

Embarking on Your Carnivore Diet Journey: Encouragement for Success

Embarking on a new dietary journey can be a daunting task, especially when it involves a radical shift like adopting the Carnivore Diet. However, for those who are curious and motivated to explore this unique approach to nutrition, there are several sources of encouragement and tips to set you on the path to success.

1. Educate Yourself

Before diving into any diet, it's essential to arm yourself with knowledge. Learn about the principles and science behind the Carnivore Diet. Understanding why and how it works can boost your confidence and commitment.

2. Start Slowly

Transitioning to a Carnivore Diet doesn't have to be an all-or-nothing endeavor. You can ease into it by gradually reducing plant-based foods from your meals. This gradual approach can make the adjustment more manageable.

3. Embrace Variety in Animal-Based Foods

While it may seem that the Carnivore Diet is limited to just meat, there's actually a wide variety of animal-based foods you can enjoy. Experiment with different cuts of meat, seafood, and organ meats to keep your meals interesting and nutritionally diverse.

4. Listen to Your Body

Pay attention to how your body responds to the diet. Everyone is unique, and what works for one person may not work for another. Be open to adjusting your food choices and quantities based on your individual needs and preferences.

5. Stay Hydrated

Proper hydration is essential, regardless of your diet. Make sure you're drinking enough water to support your body's functions, especially since the Carnivore Diet can be diuretic.

6. Seek Support

Joining online communities or forums dedicated to the Carnivore Diet can provide you with valuable support, advice, and a sense of community. Sharing your experiences and learning from others can be incredibly motivating.

7. Monitor Your Progress

Keep track of your progress, not just in terms of weight loss but also in terms of how you feel physically and mentally. Document any improvements in energy levels, mood, and overall well-being.

8. Be Patient and Persistent

Like any significant lifestyle change, adopting the Carnivore Diet may come with challenges. There may be moments of doubt or difficulty. Remember that progress takes time, and setbacks are a natural part of the journey. Stay persistent and committed to your goals.

9. Consult a Healthcare Professional

Before making any drastic changes to your diet, it's crucial to consult with a healthcare professional or a registered dietitian. They can provide personalized guidance and ensure that the Carnivore Diet is safe and appropriate for your specific health needs.

10. Enjoy the Process

Lastly, remember that your dietary journey should ultimately be a positive and enjoyable experience. Embrace the flavors and benefits of the foods you choose to eat. Celebrate your successes, no matter how small, and find joy in the process of improving your health.

Embarking on the Carnivore Diet journey can be a rewarding and transformative experience, but it's essential to approach it with knowledge, patience, and a commitment to your well-being. Remember that everyone's path is unique, and the most important thing is to prioritize your health and happiness.

The Crucial Reminder: Importance of a Well-Balanced Diet

While exploring specialized diets like the Carnivore Diet can be intriguing and potentially beneficial for some, it's essential to maintain a broader perspective on nutrition and the importance of a well-balanced diet that suits individual needs and preferences.

1. Nutritional Diversity

A well-balanced diet emphasizes the consumption of a wide range of foods, including fruits, vegetables, whole grains, lean proteins, and healthy fats. This diversity ensures that your body receives a spectrum of essential nutrients, vitamins, and minerals necessary for optimal health.

2. Long-Term Sustainability

The sustainability of a diet is a critical factor to consider. While some diets may yield short-term results, they may not be sustainable in the long run. A well-balanced diet is one that you can maintain over time, promoting not only weight management but also overall health and well-being.

3. Individual Needs

Each person's nutritional needs are unique. Factors such as age, activity level, and medical conditions can significantly influence dietary requirements. A well-balanced diet can be tailored to meet these specific needs, ensuring that you're getting the right nutrients to support your health.

4. Disease Prevention

Research consistently shows that a balanced diet rich in fruits, vegetables, and whole grains can help reduce the risk of chronic diseases such as heart disease, diabetes, and certain types of cancer. These foods provide vital antioxidants and fiber that contribute to overall well-being.

5. Enjoyment and Satisfaction

Food is not just about sustenance; it's also about enjoyment. A well-balanced diet allows for a variety of flavors and culinary experiences, making eating a pleasurable activity. This can contribute to a positive relationship with food.

6. Flexibility

Unlike highly restrictive diets, a well-balanced diet allows for flexibility and occasional indulgences. This flexibility can prevent feelings of deprivation and promote a healthier attitude towards food.

7. Holistic Health

A well-balanced diet aligns with the principles of holistic health, considering not only physical well-being but also mental and emotional health. Nourishing your body with a variety of nutrients can positively impact your overall quality of life.